D1632379

SUPER FOOD

BEETROOT

BLOOMSBURY

LONDON • OXFORD • NEW YORK • NEW DELHI • SYDNEY

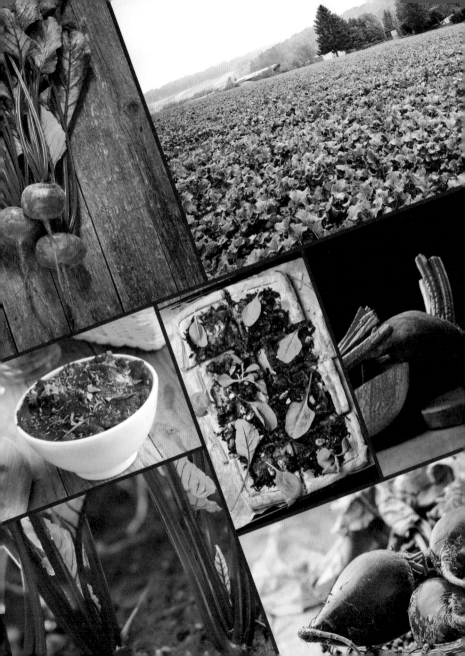

CONTENTS

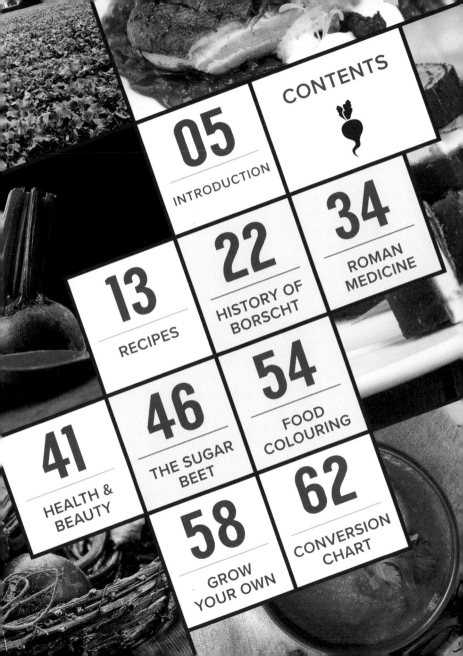

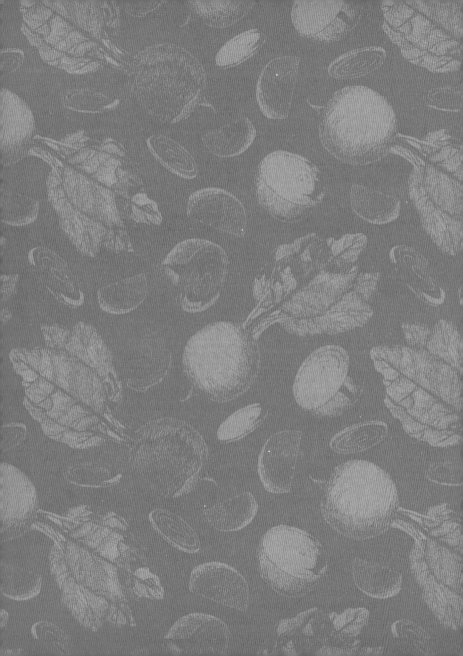

INTRODUCTION

'The beet is the most intense
of vegetables. The radish,
admittedly, is the more
feverish, but the fire of the
radish is a cold fire, the fire
of discontent not passion.
Tomatoes are lusty enough,
yet there runs through
tomatoes an undercurrent
of frivolity. Beets are
deadly serious.'

Tom Robbins
Jitterbug Perfume (2001)

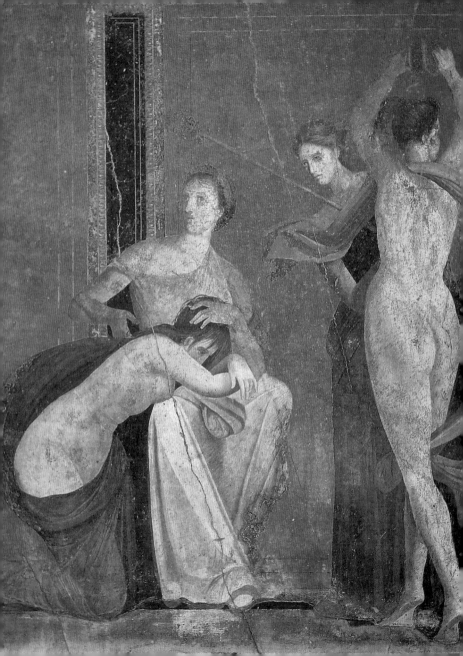

HISTORY

Beetroot (*beta vulgaris*) is the domesticated descendant of wild sea beet. The oldest evidence for its domestication dates back to Neolithic times and it was undoubtedly among the first green leafy plants to be collected and eaten by humans.

Assyrian texts tell of beetroot growing in the Hanging Gardens at Babylon, while beetroot remains dating back 5,000 years were found in excavations at Thebes. The ancient Greeks held beetroot in high esteem and included it in offerings to the sun god Apollo in his temple at Delphi, reckoning it worth its own weight in silver. Hippocrates used the leaves for binding wounds, while the Romans cultivated it for medicinal purposes – again, at this point the leaves were probably used more than the root. The Roman writer Apicius, who collated one of the first cookbooks in human history, included beetroot in recipes for stock to be used for laxative purposes. Beetroot is included in other recipes dressed with oil, vinegar and mustard, and it is assumed that the leaves were being consumed rather than the root.

The Romans regarded beetroot as an aphrodisiac and images of beetroots are found on the walls of the brothel at Pompeii. This connotation persisted and the expression 'to take favours in the beetroot fields' was a term for visiting prostitutes in the early 20th century, and was reputedly still being used by Field Marshall Montgomery during the Second World War as a suggestion to his troops. There is some justification to this perception however, as beetroots contain boron, which stimulates hormones.

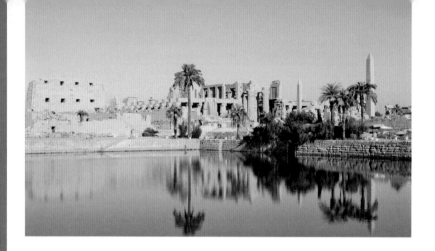

Through the Middle Ages beetroot was known as Roman beet and grown in herb gardens, again mostly for medicinal purposes. Beetroot then did not look like our modern vegetable. The Romans were familiar with a beetroot which was black and white, while the ancient form of the beetroot was long and thin like a carrot. We are more used to the modern red and round form which didn't appear until the 16th and 17th centuries, when beetroot was deliberately bred into that shape and colour, although there are still many varieties and colours of beetroot. By the 19th century the beetroot had become popular in central and eastern Europe, with the root now being used as a foodstuff,

in recipes like Ukranian borscht and Scandanavian herring salad.

> *The ancient Greeks held beetroot in high esteem and included it in offerings to the sun god Apollo in his temple at Delphi, reckoning it worth its own weight in silver.*

The Victorians mainly used beetroot to colour recipes and as a sweetener in pudding recipes. They also used it to dye hair and fabric. Victorian industrialisation increased the availability of vegetables by conserving them in jars, and after the Second World War beetroot was the most available pickled vegetable

– the main experience of beetroot until recently has been pickled in vinegar. Thankfully the beetroot has been released from its glass prison and is now being recognised for its versatility in a wide range of recipes from salad to soups.

Wild sea beet (*beta vulgaris, subsp. maritima*) is not only the ancestor of beetroot but also chard and perpetual spinach, and grows, as its name suggests, on shorelines, shingle beaches, and cliffs.

The young leaves can be eaten in the same way as chard and spinach, lightly steamed, with a little lemon juice and butter. Recently wild sea beet has been enjoying a resurgence as Michelin-starred chefs embrace wild food in their desire to add exciting new taste experiences to their menus. Food foragers are now supplying top restaurants, and sea beet leaves gathered in Wales were served to the Queen for her 80th birthday as part of *The Great British Menu*.

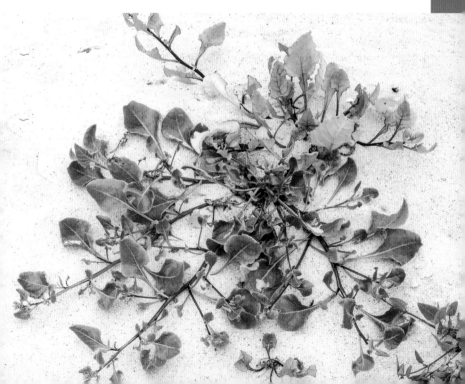

HEALTH BENEFITS

Beetroots are highly nutritious and are a rich source of vitamins and minerals including Vitamin C, potassium, magnesium, manganese, and folic acid, essential for reducing the risk of birth defects. The leafy tops are an excellent source of nutrients too including protein, zinc, iron and calcium.

For thousands of years beetroots have been used for medicinal purposes. The ancient physicians often used them in remedies for digestive complaints and fevers, and they had the right idea – beetroots contain a betacyanin called betanin, a powerful agent thought to help fight some kinds of cancer. Betanin stimulates the detoxification processes of the liver and cleanses the digestive system. It is the betanin that gives the beetroot its deep purple colour. Beetroots also contain glutamine, an amino acid which helps with digestion and boosts the immune system.

Your heart loves beetroot too. A study conducted at Queen Mary University of London in 2010 tested the effects of beetroot juice on a group of test patients, and the results showed a clear reduction in blood pressure. This is attributed to the presence of nitrates in the beetroot, which relax blood vessels thus warding off stroke and heart disease. Blood flow to the brain is also improved which may fight off dementia.

The increased nitrates may also improve sporting performance by increasing efficiency in the amount of oxygen an athlete needs to use. Many Olympic athletes now regularly drink a glass of beet juice a day when competing in an effort to acheive greater stamina

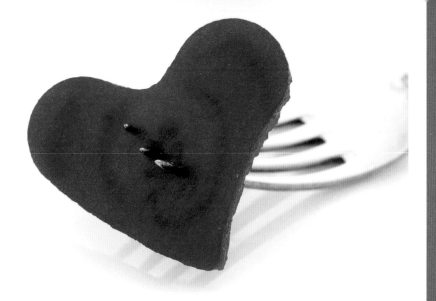

and speed. Studies support their theory: drinking the juice improved performance by 11 seconds in a 4 km bicycle time trial carried out at Exeter University in 2011.

Beetroot has a sugar content of around 10%, higher than all other vegetables, however this is a slow-release sugar which avoids spikes in blood sugar. The sweetness makes it possible to eat raw beetroot, and this means you get the full benefits of the nutrients which may be damaged in the cooking process.

Beetroots are high in fibre, which helps bowel function, preventing constipation, and also helps lower cholesterol. This fibre also increases antioxidant enzymes and white blood cells which fight abnormal cells. It can help with diabetes too as it contains an antioxidant which lowers glucose levels in the blood.

They are also virtually calorie and fat-free, so there is no need to worry about your waistline!

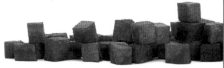

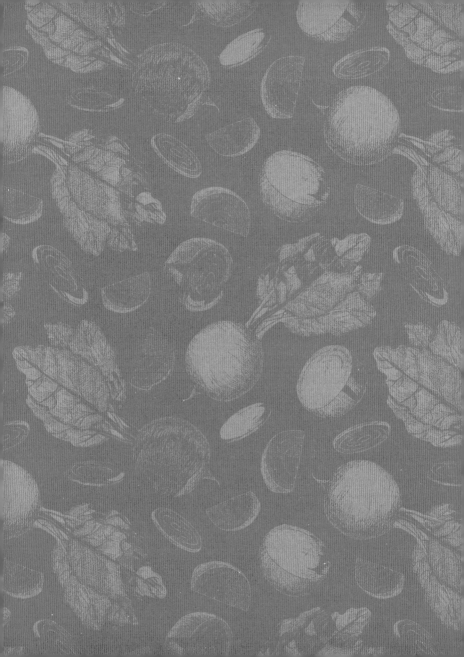

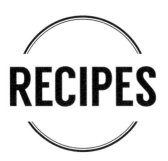

RECIPES

Recipe: Aliter ad ventrem
(Another laxative)
'Scrub and wash bundles of beets
by rubbing them with a little soda.
Tie them in individual bundles, put
into water to be cooked, when done
season with reduced must or raisin
wine and cumin, sprinkle with pepper,
add a little oil, and when hot, crush
polypody and nuts with broth, add this
to the red-hot pan, incorporating it
with the beets, take off the fire quickly
and serve.'

Apicius
De re coquinaria,
1st century AD

SERVES: **2**
PREPARATION: **5 MINUTES**

BREAKFAST SMOOTHIES

Beetroot is excellent for your digestion. Try these tasty smoothie recipes to cleanse your system and give you a great energy boost at the start of the day.

BLUEBERRY & MINT

INGREDIENTS

- 1 raw beetroot, peeled and grated
- 1 heaped tbsp chopped mint
- 1 tbsp agave syrup
- a small handful of blueberries (you can use frozen ones)
- 250ml almond milk

This bright pink smoothie combines beetroot with fresh mint and blueberries bursting with antioxidants. Place all the ingredients in a blender and whizz until fully combined. Pour into a glass and enjoy!

ORANGE, CARROT & GINGER

INGREDIENTS

- 1 raw beetroot, peeled and grated
- 200ml orange juice
- a thumb-sized piece of ginger
- ½ carrot, peeled and chopped

Fresh ginger root gives a kick to this recipe while the orange juice provides Vitamin C to boost the immune system. Blend together as above, adding more water or juice as needed to achieve the right consistency.

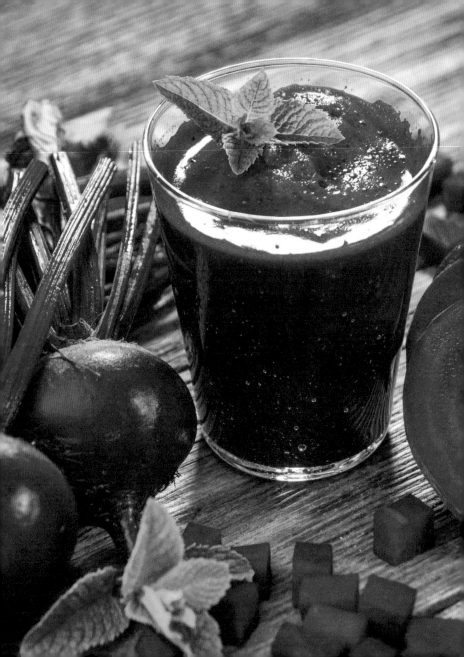

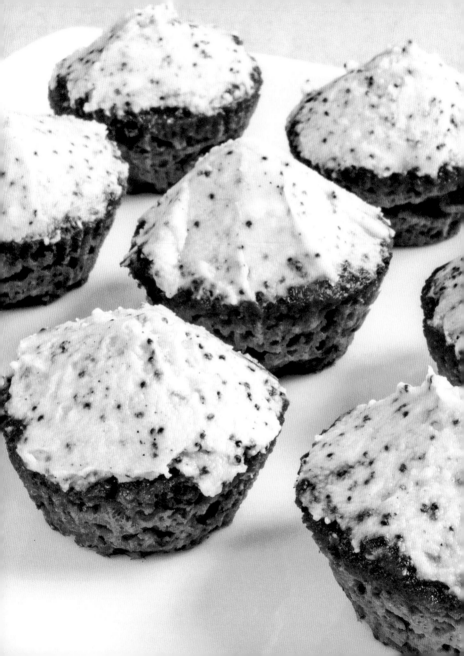

MAKES: 12 CUPCAKES
PREPARATION: 10 MINUTES
COOKING TIME: 20 MINUTES

MINI
CUPCAKES

These delicious velvety cupcakes are gorgeous to look at as well as delicious to eat.

INGREDIENTS

For the cupcakes:

- 125g plain flour
- 125g caster sugar
- 20g cocoa powder
- 1 tsp baking powder
- 2 eggs
- 100ml almond oil
- 100g cooked beetroot, finely grated

For the topping:

- 200g icing sugar
- 20g butter
- 50g cream cheese
- ½ tsp vanilla essence
- 20g chia seeds

METHOD

Preheat oven to 180°C/350°F/gas 4.

Place the flour, sugar, cocoa powder and baking powder in a mixing bowl and stir well. Beat together the eggs, almond oil and grated beetroot and add to the dry mix.

Pour into 12 cupcake cases in a baking tray. Bake for 20 minutes or until a knife comes out clean. Leave to cool.

Mix together the icing sugar, butter, cream cheese and vanilla essence until they form a smooth paste. Stir in the chia seeds and decorate your cupcakes with the topping.

SERVES: 4
PREPARATION: 10 MINUTES

BEETROOT LEAVES WITH OLIVE OIL & GARLIC

The leaves of beetroot are among the most popular green vegetables in the Puglia region of Italy. The addition of garlic and chilli balances the slightly bitter taste of the leaves, resulting in a tasty dish which can accompany a main, or be served as a starter with croutons.

💡 TOP TIP

If you can get hold of wild sea beet leaves why not try something more unusual?

INGREDIENTS

- 500g beetroot leaves
- 2 tbsp olive oil
- 1 clove of garlic
- 1 red chilli
- 1 tbsp lemon juice
- salt and freshly ground black pepper

METHOD

Steam the beetroot leaves until they wilt and are tender (around five minutes).

Heat the olive oil in a large pan or wok and gently sauté the garlic and chilli. Add the lemon juice, salt and pepper and the beetroot leaves. Do not drain the leaves too thoroughly as the water will aid the cooking process.

Stir thoroughly so the leaves pick up all the delicious flavours of the garlic, chilli and lemon, and serve immediately.

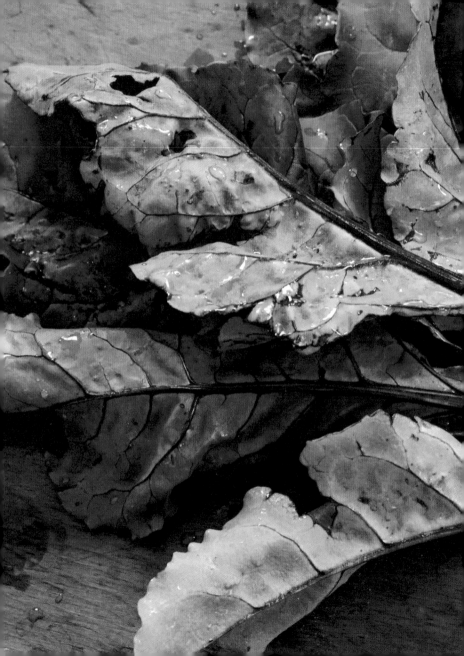

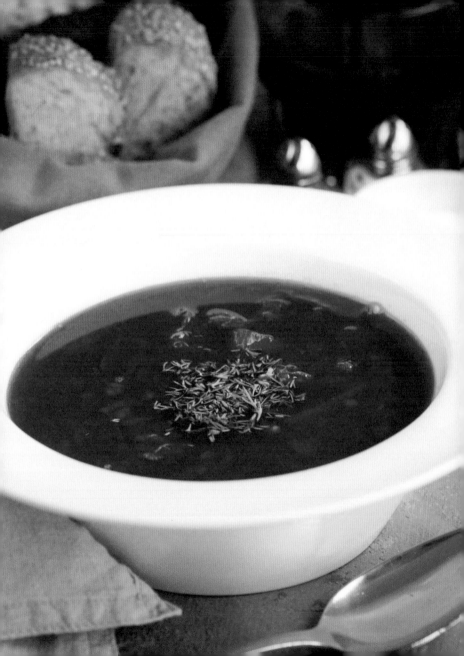

BORSCHT

SERVES: **2**
PREPARATION: **20 MINUTES**
COOKING TIME: **1 HOUR**

The famous traditional recipe from Eastern Europe, this deep purple soup has been at the heart of traditional Slavic family cooking for centuries.

INGREDIENTS

- 1 raw beetroot (approx. 200g)
- 200g red cabbage
- 1 large onion
- 1 carrot
- 1 medium sized potato
- 2 cloves garlic
- 20g butter
- 600ml beef or chicken stock
- 1 tbsp cider vinegar
- 1 tbsp tomato purée
- 1 tsp brown sugar
- ½ tsp allspice (ground)
- a bay leaf
- salt and freshly ground black pepper
- sour cream to serve

METHOD

Peel and grate the beetroot and finely chop the cabbage, onion and carrot. Peel the potato and cut into small cubes.

Melt the butter and sauté the onions and carrot until soft. Add the garlic and cook for a further minute.

Add the potato, cabbage and beetroot and stir thoroughly to coat with the flavours. Pour in the stock and bring to a gentle simmer. Add the vinegar, tomato purée, sugar, allspice and bay leaf. Season to taste.

Simmer for an hour, topping up with stock if needed. Season and serve with a dollop of sour cream.

You can blend this soup into a velvety deep purple, or leave it as it is; it's delicious either way.

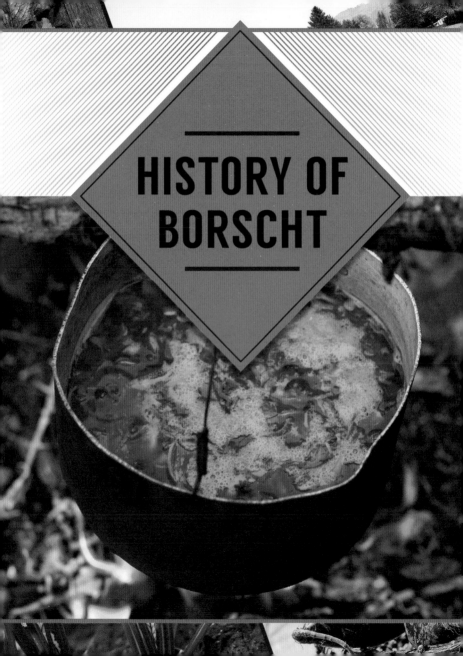

HISTORY OF
BORSCHT

The first record of a soup made with beetroot comes from the Roman gourmet Apicius, who, in his cookbook *De re coquinaria*, attributes this recipe to Marcus Terentius Varro (116–27 BC):

'Varro beets, that is, black ones of which the roots must be cleaned well, cook them with mead and a little salt and oil; boil them down in this liquor so that the roots are saturated thereby; the liquid itself is good drinking. It is also nice to cook a chicken in with them.'

This recipe is the precursor of the most famous beetroot soup of today, Russian borscht. Or is it Ukranian borsch? Each country fiercely lays claim to this soup, which has become symbolic of family and country, as recipes are passed down through the generations, surviving historical and political upheavals. It is generally accepted now that the origins of borscht are in Ukraine, although there are numerous regional variations. More versions of the soup are found throughout Eastern Europe though, from Polish *barzszc* to Lithuanian *barščiai*, each

using different ingredients and passionately claiming this soup as part of their national cuisine. With the intertwined history of Eastern European countries and the movement of their people there is no certainty as to who borscht really belongs to, but versions are lovingly created in kitchens from Odessa and Warsaw to Brooklyn, USA, with recipes handed down through the centuries, and stories to accompany them.

In 14th century Ukraine the original form of borscht was cooked using the common hogweed (the Slav word for this is *borshchevik*). In the subsistence-based peasant life hogweed was a common and hardy plant, with leaves being eaten raw and the roots boiled. It was an essential component of Slavic cookery for hundreds of years, a poor man's meal gleaned from the frozen land. But as time went on it became the dish of all Slavs, rich and poor, with variations denoting status. Meat could be added, either for guests or simply because you could afford it. At some point beetroot replaced this wild ingredient and the famous deep-red soup was born.

There is however another popular story which claims that the first borscht was cooked during the Russo–Turkish wars of the 17th century. In 1637 thousands of Cossacks laid siege to the Turkish-held Azov fortress in Southern Russia. To address the issue of feeding so many men a huge stew was thrown together consisting of anything edible that could be found, and the resulting mix was so popular that the name 'borshch' was coined for it.

There is no consistent and accepted recipe for borscht, as each generation passes on its own version, and claims it is the best and only one! The basic ingredient

> *Versions are lovingly created in kitchens from Odessa and Warsaw to Brooklyn, USA, with recipes handed down through the centuries, and stories to accompany them.*

of course is the beetroot, and most recipes include combinations of vegetables such as carrots, onions, red peppers, cabbages, potatoes and tomatoes. Many recipes now use beef stock but originally this would have been a meat-free recipe apart from on special occasions. In Poland two versions are served, a meat-free one for the feast on Christmas Eve, and a meat one for Easter. There are heated debates over how to make the perfect version; some are horrified by the idea of, for example, adding leeks, or vinegar, whilst others insist upon it. The Romanian version adds *bors*, a fermented wheat bran, whilst the Russian and Polish versions might use *kvass*, a fermented beet juice.

Whatever the recipe, the soup was traditionally made in huge batches and kept for days, improving each day as the flavours mingled (originally borscht was eaten every day, for breakfast, lunch and dinner!). Borscht for many is synonymous with their culture and feeling of identity, and the familiar rich smell evokes for some the wide open plains and frozen steppes of Eastern Europe, for others the long-gone Soviet Union. For all, though, this amazing and historical soup symbolises home: for those still living in their native lands a warm welcome to strangers, and for exiles a feeling of belonging and identity.

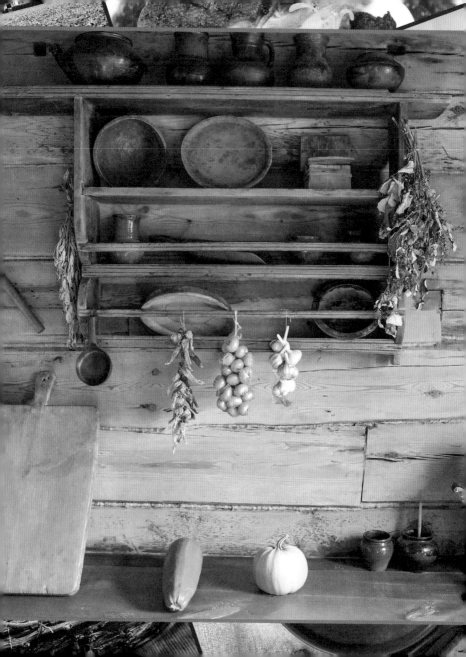

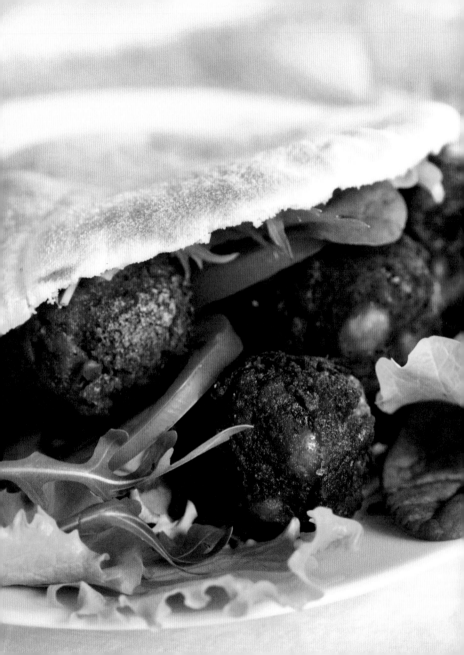

FALAFEL

MAKES: 12 FALAFEL
PREPARATION: 10 MINUTES
COOKING TIME: 25 MINUTES

(V)

This quick and easy falafel recipe makes a delicious lunchtime snack served with warm pitta bread and a yoghurt dip.

INGREDIENTS

For the falafel:

- 1 tbsp sesame oil
- 1 onion
- 2 cloves garlic
- 2 tsp ground cumin
- 250g cooked beetroot, grated
- 400g chickpeas
- a handful of coriander leaves
- 125g breadcrumbs
- 1 tbsp tahini paste
- 1 egg, beaten
- salt and freshly ground black pepper

For the yoghurt dip:

- 200g yoghurt
- 1 clove garlic
- juice of 1 lemon

METHOD

Pre-heat oven to 180°C/350°F/gas mark 4.

Chop the onion and garlic. Heat the sesame oil in a pan and sauté the onion until translucent. Add the garlic and cumin and cook for another minute.

In a food processor combine the onion mix with the grated beetroot, chickpeas, coriander leaves, breadcrumbs, tahini paste and egg. Season to taste.

Roll into balls and place on a non-stick baking tray or parchment. Bake for 20–25 minutes until crisp and hot.

To make the yoghurt dip, crush the garlic and add to the yoghurt with the lemon juice and a pinch of salt. Mix thoroughly and refrigerate until needed. Serve the falafel in warmed pitta bread with a mixed salad and the yoghurt dip.

RISOTTO

SERVES: **2**
PREPARATION: **10 MINUTES**
COOKING TIME: **20 MINUTES**

A classic recipe with a twist. Adding beetroot to risotto provides you with all the benefits of its healthy nutrients, and gives the dish an amazing deep red colour.

INGREDIENTS

- 30g butter
- 1 tbsp olive oil
- 3 shallots, peeled and chopped finely
- 2 garlic cloves, peeled and chopped finely
- 175g arborio risotto rice
- 500ml vegetable stock
- 250g cooked beetroot
- 75ml white wine
- juice of ½ lemon
- 50g parmesan
- 1 tsp freshly chopped thyme
- salt and freshly ground black pepper

To serve:

- 100g ricotta cheese, torn into pieces
- rocket leaves
- balsamic vinegar

METHOD

Melt the butter in a pan and add the olive oil. Sauté the shallots gently until translucent. Add the garlic and cook for a further minute.

Add the rice and stir for a minute until the grains are fully coated and have absorbed the butter. Now gradually add the stock, a ladleful at a time, waiting until the liquid is absorbed before adding the next ladleful.

Cut the beetroot into pieces and blend until it forms a purée. Add water as needed to achieve the right consistency.

Once all the stock is absorbed, add the white wine, lemon juice, parmesan and thyme, and finally stir in the beetroot purée. Season to taste.

Serve with the ricotta cheese scattered on top and a rocket salad dressed with balsamic vinegar.

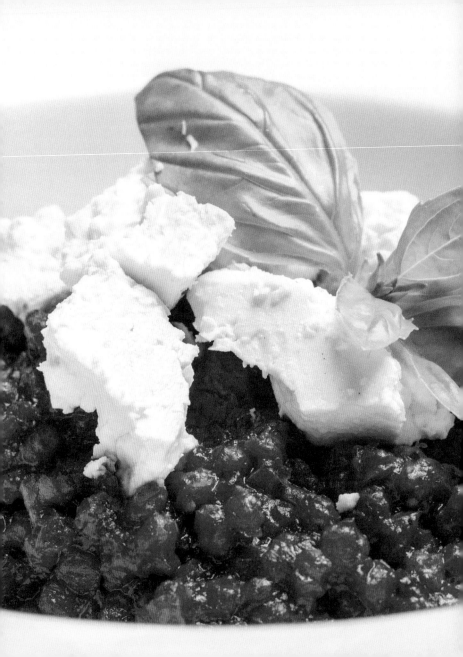

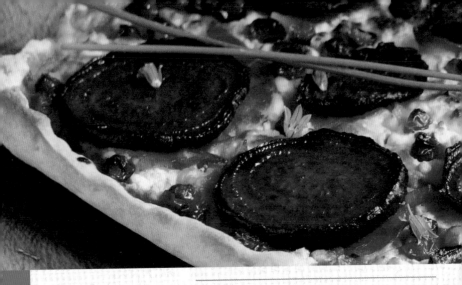

BEETROOT, GOAT'S CHEESE & THYME TART

SERVES: 4
PREPARATION: 15 MINUTES
COOKING TIME: 20 MINUTES

The sweetness of beetroot is balanced by a tangy goat's cheese in this stylish tart which makes a great starter or light lunch.

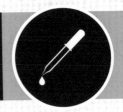

ALKALINE SOLUTIONS WILL TURN BEETROOT JUICE YELLOW. WHILE ACIDIC SOLUTIONS WILL MAKE IT PINK.

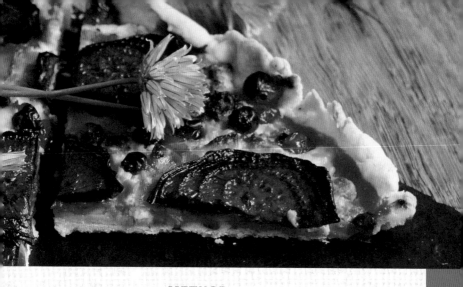

INGREDIENTS

- 2 tbsp olive oil
- 2 large red onions, finely sliced
- a small bunch of thyme leaves, chopped
- salt and freshly ground black pepper
- 250g puff pastry
- 200g cooked beetroot, sliced
- 100g goat's cheese, sliced
- rocket leaves and balsamic vinegar to serve

METHOD

Preheat oven to 200°C/400°F/gas 6.

Heat the olive oil and gently cook the onions with most of the thyme until soft and translucent. Season to taste. Reserve the remaining thyme to scatter on top.

Roll out the puff pastry, prick all over with a fork and bake for ten minutes. Gently push the middle down if it has risen in the oven, or you can use ceramic baking beans to prevent it rising.

Spread the onion mixture over the puff pastry base and arrange the slices of beetroot and goat's cheese on top. Scatter over the remaining thyme leaves.

Bake in the oven for 20 minutes or until the pastry is golden-brown. Serve with the rocket and balsamic vinegar salad.

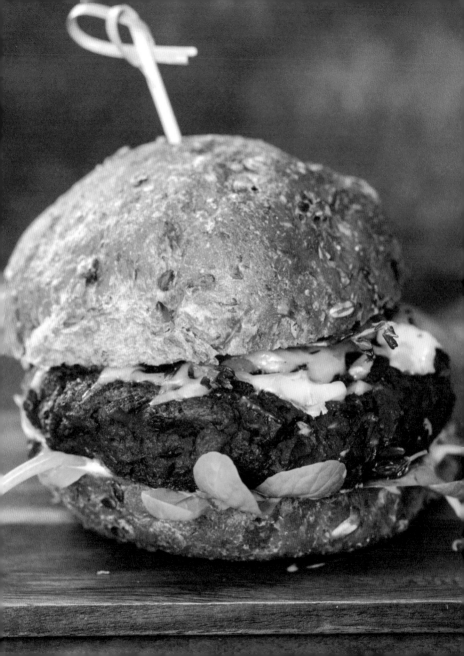

SERVES: 4
PREPARATION: 20 MINUTES
COOKING TIME: 30 MINUTES

BURGER

The ultimate veggie burger. Lentils are full of nutrients and healthy fibre while the beetroot adds sweetness.

INGREDIENTS

- 100g puy lentils
- 500ml chicken or vegetable stock
- 1 onion
- 1 tbsp olive oil
- 2 cloves of garlic
- 2 cooked beetroot, grated
- 1 egg, beaten
- 100g breadcrumbs
- 1 tsp coriander
- 2 tsp smoked paprika
- 1 tsp cumin
- ½ tsp thyme
- 1 tsp chilli powder
- salt and freshly ground black pepper
- 4 large field mushrooms
- burger bun
- Stilton
- a little gem lettuce

METHOD

Preheat oven to 180°C/350°F/gas 4.

Place the lentils in the stock and simmer until soft. Meanwhile sauté the onion gently in the olive oil until translucent, stirring frequently. Add the chopped garlic and cook for a further minute.

Once the lentils are soft, place in a food processor and blend with the onion mix, grated beetroot, egg, lentils, breadcrumbs, herbs and spices and season to taste.

Shape the mix into burgers on a flour-covered board, and dust the burgers lightly with flour. Place on a greased baking tray. Drizzle the field mushrooms with olive oil and place on a baking tray in the oven at the same time.

Cook for half an hour until the burgers are crispy and hot and the mushrooms soft. Turn the burgers half way through cooking.

Place each burger in a bun, put a mushroom on each and top with Stilton. Serve with little gem lettuce.

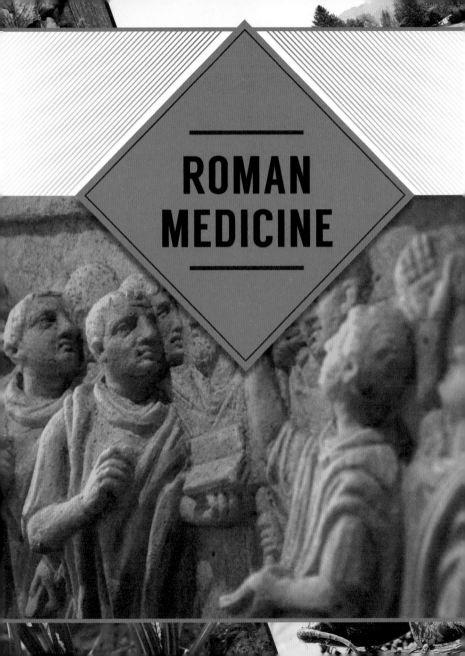

ROMAN MEDICINE

The Roman writer Pliny the Elder (23–79 AD) suggested many interesting medicinal uses for beetroot, in his scientific work *Natural History*, which became a standard reference work until the Middle Ages.

After a career in the military Pliny spent his retirement studying and writing. On the subject of beetroot he suggested the following uses:

'Nor are the two varieties of the beet without their remedial properties. The root of either white or black beet, if hung by a string, fresh-gathered, and softened with water, is said to be efficacious for the stings of serpents. White beet, boiled and eaten with raw garlic, is taken for tapeworm; the root, too, of the black kind, similarly boiled in water, removes porrigo; indeed, it is generally stated that the black beet is the more efficacious of the two. The juice of black beet is good for inveterate head-aches and

> *The root of either white or black beet … is said to be efficacious for the stings of serpents.*

vertigo, and injected into the ears, it stops singing in those organs. It is a diuretic, also, and employed in injections is a cure for dysentery and jaundice.

This juice, used as a liniment, allays tooth-ache, and is good for the stings of serpents; but due care must be taken that it is extracted from this root only. A decoction, too, of beet-root is a remedy for chilblains.

A liniment of white beet-root applied to the forehead, arrests defluxions of the eyes, and mixed up with a little alum it is an excellent remedy for erysipelas. Beaten up, and applied without oil, it is a cure for excoriations. In the same way, too, it is good for pimples and eruptions. Boiled, it is applied topically to spreading ulcers, and in a raw state it is employed in cases of alopecy, and running ulcers of the head. The juice, injected with honey into the nostrils, has the effect of clearing the head. Beet-root is boiled with lentils and vinegar, for the purpose of relaxing the bowels; if it is boiled, however, some time longer, it will have the effect of arresting fluxes of the stomach and bowels.'
Natural History, Book XVII

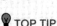

💡 TOP TIP

For beetroot syrup, place a small chopped beetroot in 200ml water with 1½ tsp sugar and simmer for 20 minutes. Take the beetroot out and you are left with around 75ml syrup.

INGREDIENTS

For the macaroons:

- 200g icing sugar
- 125g ground almonds
- 3 egg whites
- ½ tsp cream of tartar
- 2 tbsp caster sugar
- 75ml beetroot syrup (see Top Tip)

For the cream:

- 100ml double cream
- 2 tsp beetroot syrup

MACAROONS WITH BEETROOT CREAM

Beetroots have been used as a food colourant in puddings for centuries. Here they add a beautiful pink colour to the classic macaroon.

METHOD

Preheat the oven to 160°C/325°F/gas 3.

Sift the icing sugar into a bowl and mix in the ground almonds. Whisk the egg with the cream of tartar and caster sugar until it forms peaks. Gently fold in the icing sugar and almonds, and finally stir through the beetroot syrup, reserving a couple of teaspoons for the cream.

Line a baking tray with greaseproof paper and pipe the macaroon mixture into flat circles around 5cm wide. Cook for around ten minutes. Set aside to cool while you make the cream.

Whisk the cream until it forms peaks and fold in the remaining beetroot syrup.

Sandwich the macaroons together with the beetroot cream filling and leave to chill before serving.

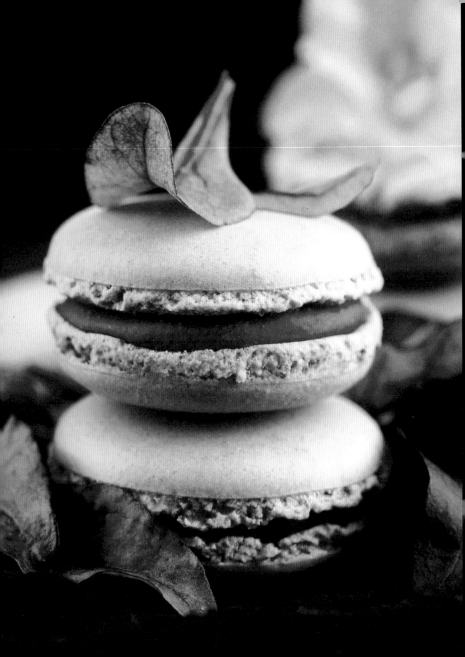

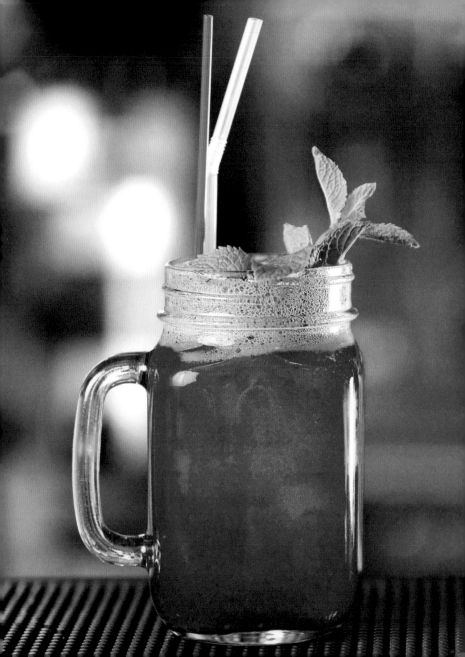

SERVES: **2**
PREPARATION: **5 MINUTES**

BEETROOT-
INFUSED GIN

Beetroot can be used to make a sweet pink wine, but that can take a few months, so instead, try this simple recipe for a beetroot-infused gin.

INGREDIENTS

- 1 small uncooked beet, peeled and chopped into pieces
- 50ml gin
- ½ tsp sugar
- a handful of fresh mint leaves, to serve

METHOD

Place the beetroot pieces into a glass jar with the gin and sugar and leave overnight in a cool, dark place. Strain the liquid and keep refrigerated.

Place a generous scoop of ice cubes in a glass and pour the gin over. Add tonic water and the mint leaves and leave to steep for a few minutes.

BEETROOT HAS A SUGAR CONTENT OF AROUND 10%, WHICH IS HIGHER THAN ALL OTHER VEGETABLES, BUT IT IS A HEALTHY, SLOW-RELEASE SUGAR.

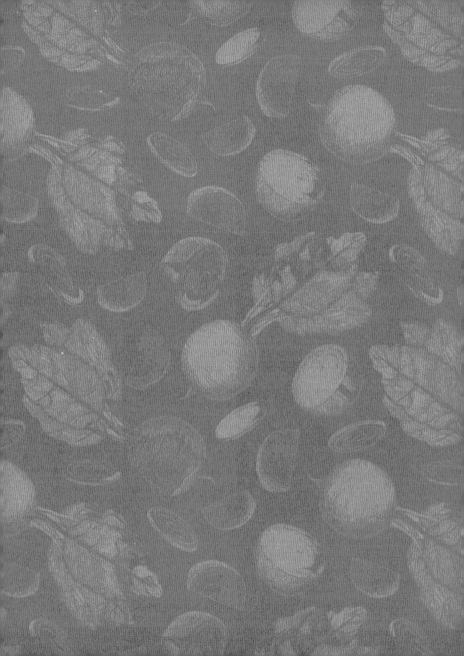

HEALTH & BEAUTY

'[Beetroot] is not an inspiring vegetable, unless you have a medieval passion for highly coloured food. With all that purple juice bleeding out at the tiniest opportunity, a cook may reasonably feel that beetroot has taken over the kitchen and is far too bossy a vegetable. I have never heard anyone claim it as their favourite.'

Jane Grigson's
Vegetable book, 1978

FACIAL TREATMENTS

The antioxidants in beetroot juice boost collagen production thus keeping your skin smooth, while beetroot's antibacterial properties and Vitamin C clean and brighten your skin.

INGREDIENTS

- 1 tbsp beetroot juice (see opposite)
- 1 tbsp yoghurt
- 1 tsp almond oil

CLEANSING FACE MASK

Mix the ingredients well and apply to your face. Relax and leave the mask on for 20 minutes before gently rinsing off.

INGREDIENTS

- 1 tbsp beetroot juice
- 1 tbsp lemon juice

SKIN-BRIGHTENING TREATMENT

For a skin-brightening mask for dull skin, mix the beetroot juice and lemon juice together. Sweep the lotion over your face with cotton wool pads and leave for 20 minutes before rinsing off.

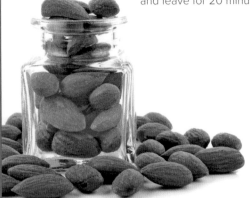

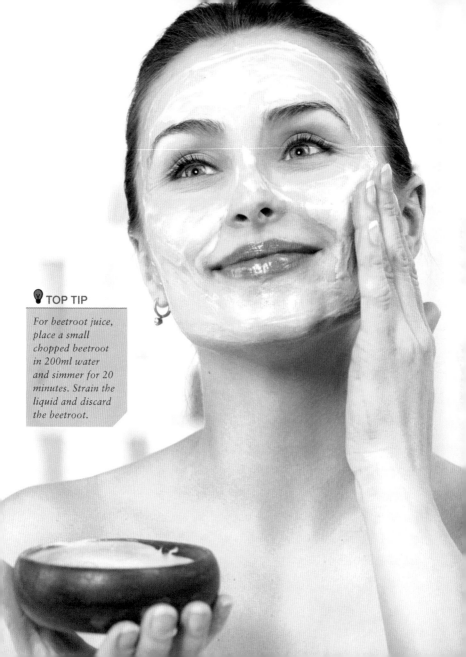

💡 TOP TIP

For beetroot juice, place a small chopped beetroot in 200ml water and simmer for 20 minutes. Strain the liquid and discard the beetroot.

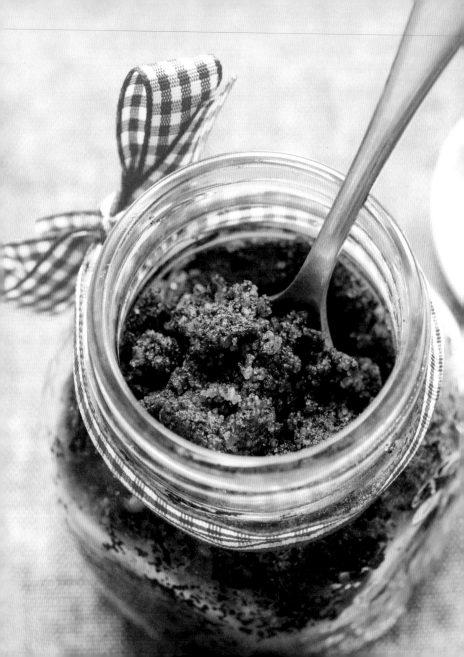

LIP TREATMENT

For an exfoliating lip treatment, try this natural scrub recipe using brown sugar. The coconut oil will moisturise your lips while the beetroot juice cleans and brightens them.

METHOD

Soften the coconut oil and blend with the honey until fully combined. Stir in the brown sugar, then add the beetroot juice and lemon juice.

Put the mixture into a small jar and allow it to harden in the fridge. When you are ready to use it let it warm up for a few minutes, then massage your home-made scrub gently onto your lips for a smooth clean feeling. Wash off with warm water.

INGREDIENTS

- 1 tbsp coconut oil
- 1 tbsp honey
- 2 tsp soft brown sugar
- 1 tsp beetroot juice (see p 42)
- 1 tsp lemon

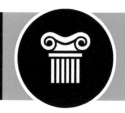

BEETROOTS HAVE A LONG ASSOCIATION WITH GLAMOUR. IT IS SAID THAT APHRODITE. THE GREEK GODDESS OF LOVE. ATE THEM TO PRESERVE HER BEAUTY.

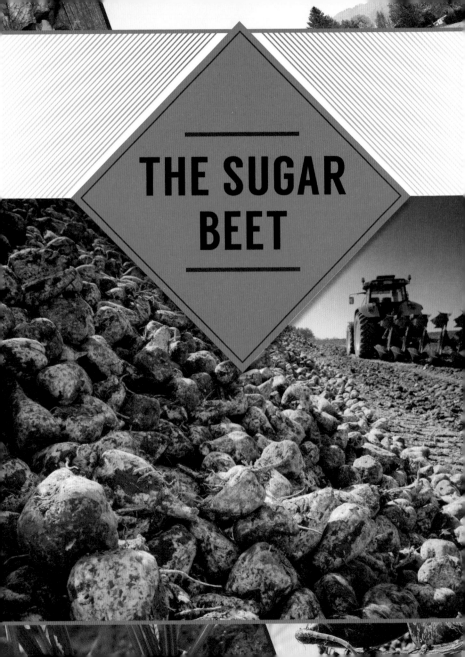

THE SUGAR
BEET

Until the 19th century Europe relied on sugar imports from sugar cane plantations in the Americas, which used slave labour. This reliance was called into question following a slave rebellion in Haiti in 1791 which led to widespread unrest across the plantations. The uprising sparked growing discomfort about the morality of slavery.

The French Republic had outlawed slavery in its constitution of 1793, and in Britain the Abolitionist movement gained a momentum which led ultimately to the abolition of slavery in 1833. Labour on the plantations now had to be paid for, and so costs went up, just as Europeans had developed a taste for sugar. Luckily there was an alternative to sugar cane ... the beetroot.

Beetroot has the highest concentration of sugar of any vegetable, and from the 16th century herbalists were extracting a sweet syrup from its swollen roots. In 1747 the German scientist Andreas Marggraf conducted an experiment to determine the sugar content of the beetroot. He sliced, dried and pulverised beet plants and extracted their juice using boiling alcohol. Using a microscope he then studied the dried crystallised juice with a microscope and demonstrated that the crystals which had formed were the same as those found in sugar cane. His results were publicised but the low amount of sugar extracted was not considered worth pursuing and the main source of sugar remained cane.

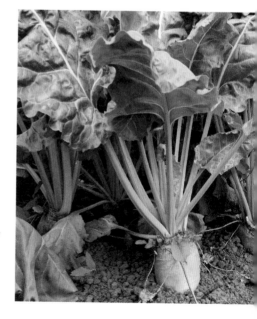

Fifty years later Marggraf's student Franz Achard carried on his work, and began to select and cultivate beets with a view to improving their sugar content. He experimented with soil conditions and growing methods until he had produced a variety of sugar beet, which he named 'White Silesian Beet', that consistently yielded high amounts of sugar.

In 1799 Achard presented Frederick William III, the King of Prussia, with a sugarloaf made from beet and requested funding for the first commercial extraction of sugar from sugar beet. In 1802 the first factory was built in Lower Silesia, followed by a larger estate built by Achard's friend Moritz Baron von Koppy. Koppy and Achard's experimentation resulted in efficient processing methods and they taught others how to grow and harvest sugar beet.

During the Napoleonic Wars of 1803–1815, French ports were blockaded by the English and the supplies of sugar from the West Indies were unable to get through. Napoleon had also tried Achard's sugarloaf and decided to support

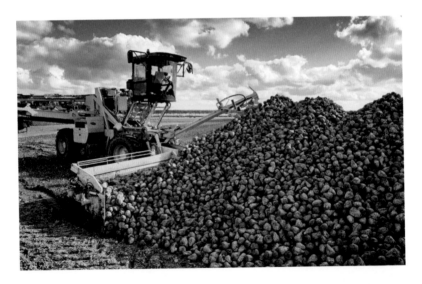

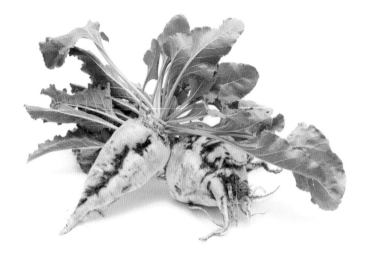

a policy of intense indigenous sugar production. In 1811 around 40 new small factories were set up across Germany and France, and although production declined after Napoleon's defeat, this period of cultivation proved that the climate of Europe was ideal for this crop.

Experimentation in sweet beets had continued, however, and by the 1830s production had increased again, with technical advances made to improve sugar extraction. Sugar was being extracted from beet across Eastern Europe, and the process eventually spread into America as German and French immigrants bought the know-how with them. During the First World War German U-boats patrolling the Atlantic threatened supplies from America to Britain, and as a result crops of sugar beet were established in Britain, and still grow today.

Today around 20% of the world's sugar is extracted from sugar beet, and around 90% of sugar consumed in Europe is grown locally. With the realisation that sugar is incredibly bad for us and the accompanying concerns over obesity, other uses for the crop are being discovered, including biofuels and other industrial products.

LIPSTAIN

💡 **TOP TIP**

To remove beetroot stains from your hands run them under cold water and then rub them with salt or baking soda.

Women have been using powdered beetroot to redden their cheeks and lips for thousands of years, and it is still used today in natural cosmetic recipes.

During the Second World War, when cosmetics were hard to come by, women used beetroot juice to stain their lips.

Try this recipe to achieve a vintage 1940s look, with this natural red-pink lipstain.

INGREDIENTS

- 1 tbsp beetroot juice (see p 42)
- 1 tbsp lemon juice
- 1 tsp olive oil

METHOD

Mix the ingredients together. The olive oil will help to moisturise your lips and the lemon juice will preserve the colour. Dab on your lips, allow to dry and repeat until you have the depth of colour you like.

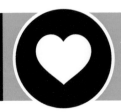

THERE IS STILL A BELIEF IN SOME CULTURES THAT IF A MAN AND A WOMAN SHARE A BEETROOT THEY WILL FALL IN LOVE.

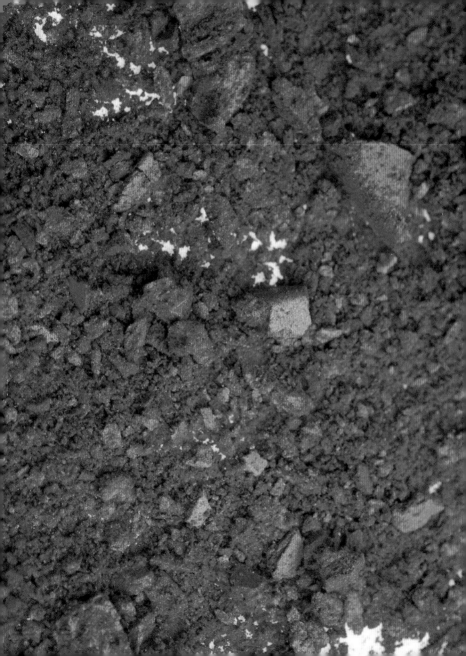

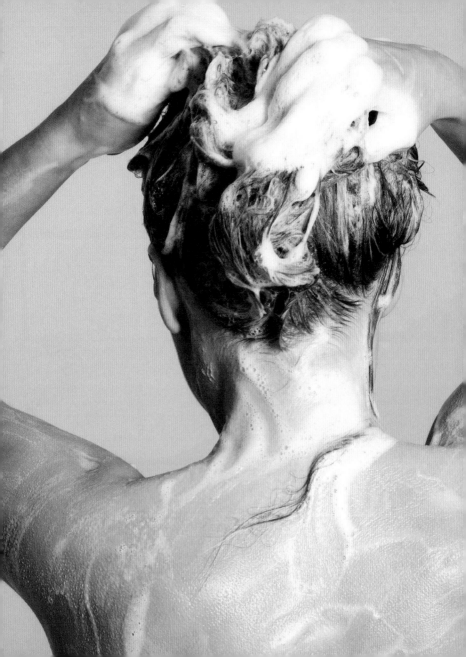

HAIR TREATMENT

Beetroot's nutrients and vitamins have many benefits for hair and scalp. They can help to stimulate hair growth, reduce hair loss, tackle dandruff and even colour your hair without the use of harsh chemicals.

HAIR LOSS

Simply drinking beetroot juice or eating the flesh has been shown to reduce hair loss by stimulating new growth. Add beets to your daily diet and see the results!

DANDRUFF TREATMENT

Boil two raw beetroots in water and gently simmer for about an hour. Turn off the heat, discard the beets and allow the water to cool. Pour the water into a clean, sterile spray bottle and keep in the fridge. Every evening for at least a week (longer if necessary), spray the scalp with the water and massage in for a few minutes.

 TOP TIP

Beetroots contain protein, calcium, iron and nutrients including manganese, potassium, Vitamin B6 and folic acid – all of which are essential for keeping your hair in great condition.

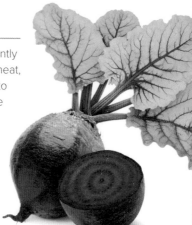

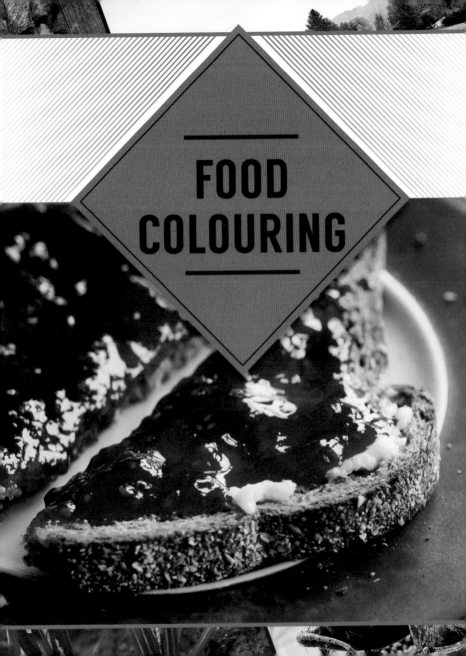

FOOD
COLOURING

Food has been coloured for thousands of years as people sought to make it more appealing and flavoursome. Beetroots were used as their rich red juice, a result of their high betanin content, was easily extracted to provide a natural colourant. Until the 19th century the leaves were also used, particularly for colouring sweets, as they produced a green dye known as beet leaf green.

During the Industrial Revolution natural dyes were replaced with synthetic colourants and even with poisonous substances. Red lead, copper sulphate, chloride and many other chemicals were used to produce brightly-coloured sweets in order to attract children. In 1858 tragedy struck in Bradford when around 200 people, including children, were poisoned, 20 fatally, after eating peppermint lozenges which accidentally contained arsenic. The so-called Bradford Sweets Poisoning led to a public outcry and a demand for action.

Regulation was clearly called for and in 1860 the Adulteration of Food and Drink Act was passed to monitor the use of colourants, although it wasn't until 1906 that artificial colours 'injurious to health' were banned. The first European Directive 'concerning the colouring matters authorized for use in foodstuffs intended for human consumption' was published in 1962 and listed only 36 permitted colourants, including number E162 – Beetroot red, betanin.

Beetroot is today widely used to colour a variety of foodstuffs from burgers, tomato paste, yoghurt, jams and soup to puddings and drinks, due to the small amount needed and the minimal flavour it adds.

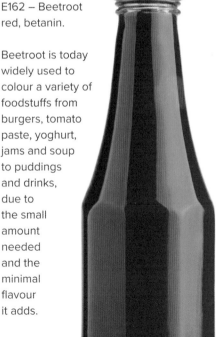

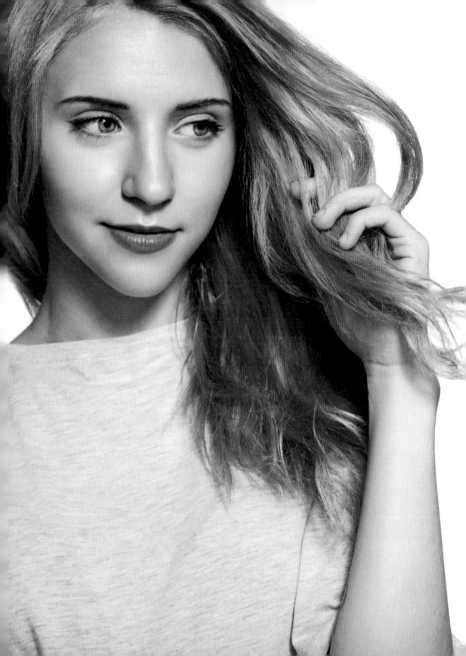

BEETROOT &
HENNA HAIR DYE

This treatment should give you a rich hair colour for roughly a week. You can play around with amounts of henna and beetroot until you have found the perfect combination for your colour and style. Just remember to wear gloves!

METHOD

Pour the juice into a bowl. Stir in the henna powder, and transfer the mixture into a clean, sterile bottle (a regular shampoo bottle is best).

Pour enough shampoo for about five washes into the clean bottle. Use a small funnel to pour the henna and beet juice mix into the same clean bottle. Shake well to combine the shampoo and beetroot juice.

Test on a small section of hair as you may have to add more shampoo or henna and beet juice mix depending on the intensity of colour you want. Leave the mixture in for one to two hours depending on how deep you want the colour and the lightness of your natural hair colour.

Rinse with warm water until the water runs clear.

 TOP TIP

A thin layer of Vaseline around your hairline and ears will prevent the dye from staining your skin. Also wrap your hair in clingfilm while you wait for it to set, to prevent dripping and to intensify the treatment.

YOU WILL NEED

- 75ml beetroot juice (see p 42)
- ½ tbsp henna powder
- a large bowl
- sulphate-free shampoo
- a small funnel
- a clean shampoo bottle
- plastic gloves

GROW YOUR OWN

Beetroots are best grown in the spring or autumn, as they like sunshine but not too much heat or dryness.

Plant your seeds in seed trays in a greenhouse or on a window-sill as beetroot does not like the cold and will not germinate if it is not warm enough. When the seedlings reach around 2cm high thin them out and keep the strongest ones.

Once the ground temperature has warmed up to above 10°C you can plant the seedlings out, but you may need to use a horticultural fleece to keep the soil warm for them in case the temperature drops again. You can also plant the seeds directly in the soil once it is warm enough and again, a fleece will help with this.

Plant the seedlings in well-prepared moist soil leaving a space of around 20cm for small beetroots. If you want them to grow larger you need to leave a bigger gap. To ensure a regular crop plant another row each month. Water them well every week,

and avoid overwatering as it will stimulate leaf growth at the expense of the roots.

You can harvest the beetroots after about eight weeks depending on how big you want them to be – they can be eaten when they reach the size of a golf ball but they will eventually reach the size of a tennis ball. Each time you sow another row you can harvest the earlier beets.

Pull them up by gently pulling on the leaves or levering out with a trowel. Remember you can eat the leaves too in the same way as spinach.

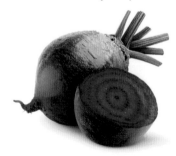

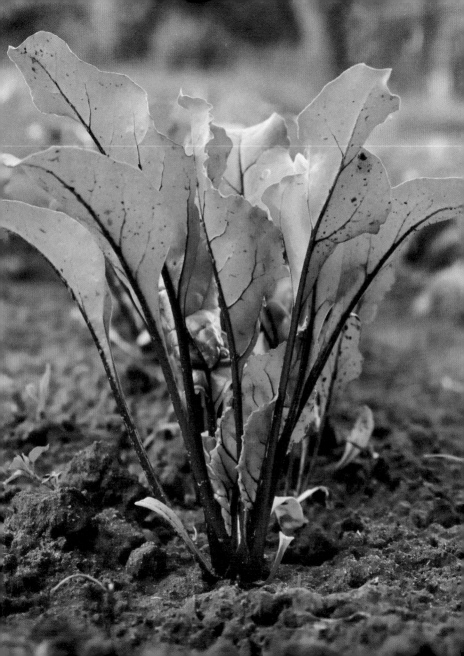

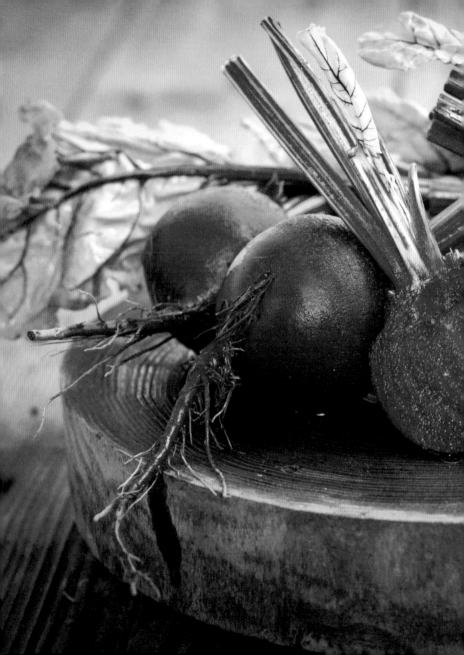

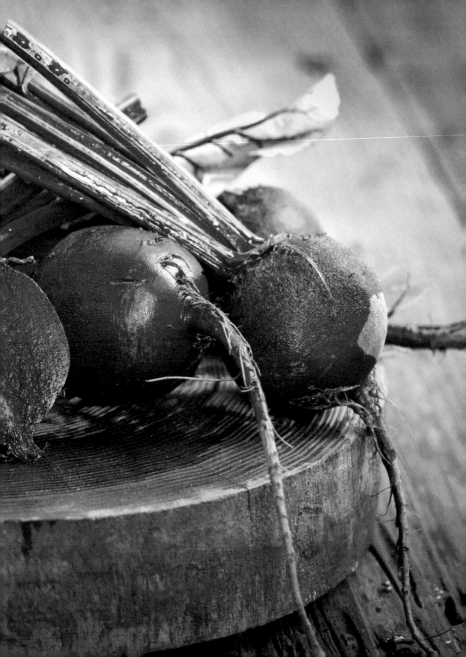

CONVERSION CHART
FOR COMMON MEASUREMENTS

LIQUIDS

15 ml	½ fl oz
25 ml	1 fl oz
50 ml	2 fl oz
75 ml	3 fl oz
100 ml	3 ½ fl oz
125 ml	4 fl oz
150 ml	¼ pint
175 ml	6 fl oz
200 ml	7 fl oz
250 ml	8 fl oz
275 ml	9 fl oz
300 ml	½ pint
325 ml	11 fl oz
350 ml	12 fl oz
375 ml	13 fl oz
400 ml	14 fl oz
450 ml	¾ pint
475 ml	16 fl oz
500 ml	17 fl oz
575 ml	18 fl oz
600 ml	1 pint
750 ml	1 ¼ pints
900 ml	1 ½ pints
1 litre	1 ¾ pints
1.2 litres	2 pints
1.5 litres	2 ½ pints
1.8 litres	3 pints
2 litres	3 ½ pints
2.5 litres	4 pints
3.6 litres	6 pints

WEIGHTS

5 g	¼ oz
15 g	½ oz
20 g	¾ oz
25 g	1 oz
50 g	2 oz
75 g	3 oz
125 g	4 oz
150 g	5 oz
175 g	6 oz
200 g	7 oz
250 g	8 oz
275 g	9 oz
300 g	10 oz
325 g	11 oz
375 g	12 oz
400 g	13 oz
425 g	14 oz
475 g	15 oz
500 g	1 lb
625 g	1 ¼ lb
750 g	1 ½ lb
875 g	1 ¾ lb
1 kg	2 lb
1.25 kg	2 ½ lb
1.5 kg	3 lb
1.75 kg	3 ½ lb
2 kg	4 lb

OVEN TEMPERATURES

110°C .... (225°F) .... gas mark ¼
120°C .... (250°F) .... gas mark ½
140°C .... (275°F) .... gas mark 1
150°C .... (300°F) .... gas mark 2
160°C .... (325°F) .... gas mark 3
180°C .... (350°F) .... gas mark 4
190°C .... (375°F) .... gas mark 5
200°C ...... (400°F) .... gas mark 6
220°C ...... (425°F) .... gas mark 7
230°C ...... (450°F) .... gas mark 8

MEASUREMENTS

5 mm .... ¼ inch
1 cm .... ½ inch
1.5 cm .... ¾ inch
2.5 cm .... 1 inch
5 cm .... 2 inches
7 cm .... 3 inches
10 cm .... 4 inches
12 cm .... 5 inches
15 cm .... 6 inches
18 cm .... 7 inches
20 cm .... 8 inches
23 cm .... 9 inches
25 cm .... 10 inches
28 cm .... 11 inches
30 cm .... 12 inches
33 cm .... 13 inches

KEY TO SYMBOLS

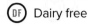 Dairy free

 Gluten free

 Vegetarian

 Vegan

A NOTE ON USING DIFFERENT OVENS

Not all ovens are the same, and the more cooking you do the better you will get to know yours. If a recipe says that you need to bake something for ten minutes or until golden brown, use your judgment as to whether it needs a few extra minutes. Conversely don't overcook food by following the timings rigidly if you think it looks ready.

As a general rule gas ovens have more uneven heat distribution so the top of the oven may be hotter than the bottom. Electric ovens tend to maintain a regular temperature throughout and distribute heat more evenly, especially fan ovens.

All the recipes in this book have been tested in an electric oven with a fan. Recommended oven temperatures are provided for electric (Celsius and Fahrenheit), and gas. If you have a fan oven then lower the electric temperature by 20°.

Bloomsbury Publishing

An imprint of Bloomsbury Publishing plc

50 Bedford Square
London
WC1B 3DP
UK

1385 Broadway
New York
NY 10018
USA

www.bloomsbury.com

BLOOMSBURY and the Diana logo are trademarks of Bloomsbury Publishing Plc

First Published in 2017

© Bloomsbury Publishing plc

Created for Bloomsbury by Plum5 Ltd

Photographs and Illustrations © Shutterstock

British Library Cataloguing-in-Publication Data

A catalogue record for this book is available from the British Library.

Library of Congress Cataloguing-in-Publication Data

A catalogue record for this book is available from the Library of Congress.

ISBN: 9781408887318

2 4 6 8 10 9 7 5 3 1

Printed in China by C&C Printing

To find out more about our authors and books visit www.bloomsbury.com.
Here you will find extracts, author interviews, details of forthcoming events
and the option to sign up for our newsletters.